15 REASONS I'M CHILDFREE

REAL Stories to Validate Your Childfree Choice

JERRA LATRICE MITCHELL

Published in the United States by Gifted With a Pen.

Proofreader: Cameron Harris (the author's nephew)
Book Cover Design by: Unique Period and Monica Steven
ISBN: 979-8-89705-972-0

TABLE OF CONTENTS

INTRODUCTION

I'll never forget my most recent international trip. While sitting in the beautifully decorated Taipei-Taoyuan International Airport in Taiwan, during my layover to Bali, Indonesia, I was approached by a man. He appeared to be in his late 50s and reminded me of a more stout version of Jet Li. When we made eye contact, he smiled, and asked, "How are you?" I replied with the standard, "I'm fine" response. I also asked how he was doing. He paused for a moment, then put emphasis on ARE (*"How **ARE** you?"*), as he sensed my response wasn't authentic.

I blinked my eyes, smiled a little, sat up straight, and thought more carefully about my answer. I responded with, "I'm grateful. Simply grateful." He smiled, and exclaimed, "That's the spirit!" His next set of questions were also intriguing and I made sure to answer them with more thought and intention.

Then, he asked me, "What's your life philosophy?" No one had ever asked me that before. I drank a bit of my tea, sat back in my chair, and cracked my knuckles before responding. I said, "I aim to live with no regrets." A simple, yet profound answer. Before I knew it, our amazing conversation had to be cut short because my connecting flight to Bali was starting to board.

That entire interaction really opened my eyes and confirmed how superficial and menial some (if not MOST) conversations are in the United States. When meeting new people, they always ask the common 3 questions during every interaction. You might be wondering what the Common 3's are. They are:

- *What do you do for a living?*
- *How many kids do you have?*
- *Are you married or in a relationship?*

These sound quite familiar, don't they? Most people don't realize these questions can be intrusive and triggering for some - especially the question about kids. I really wish our interactions were more meaningful, like the one I experienced that beautiful September afternoon in the Taipei Airport.

We live in a patriarchal society that believes everyone <u>needs</u> to create a family and "build a legacy." (*As if having a family is the only way to build a legacy, right?*) When someone chooses to go against the "norm," they're often faced with criticism and are told, "You'll regret it one day." When will some people realize not everyone desires motherhood/fatherhood? Being a parent isn't for everyone.

When I was 15 years old, my childfree choice was solidified. No matter how many times I heard, "*You're going to change your mind one day!*," I knew I would <u>never</u> get pregnant and become someone's mother. That's how self-aware I was (and still am).

In a nutshell, this book consists of 15 childfree stories. Twelve of these stories are my own, three stories are those of my childfree friends, then there's three bonus stories involving deceased childfree public figures (to dispute the "*legacy*" argument). This book is also filled with childfree quotes, fun facts, and takeaways.

Also, throughout this book, you'll see that I use the word "children" instead of "kids." In the dictionary, the word "kids" refers to a baby goat. So yeah…even though I don't want children, I still make a cognizant effort to respect them. ☺

Upon reading this book, you will feel seen, supported, and understood as a childfree person. I commend you for going against societal norms and being true to yourself. Being childfree is a valid life choice - one that you should be proud of.

Your worth is **not** defined by parenthood. It is **NOT** your sole purpose in life to become someone's mother/father. Others may experience fulfillment and happiness from having children, and that's OK. There are a myriad of things in life that bring fulfillment and joy, that don't involve starting a family.

Lastly, if you're not childfree and still decided to purchase and read this book, thank you from the bottom of my heart!

Jerra Latrice Mitchell

Childfree Fact #1
(International Childfree Day)

*Did you know International Childfree Day exists?
Yep, it's a thing!*

*International Childfree Day is observed annually on
August 1st. It was established in 1973 in the United
States by the National Alliance for Optional Parenthood
(NAOP), at the time the National Organization for
Non-Parents, under the name of Non-Parents' Day. Its sole
purpose is to recognize and celebrate people who choose not
to have children.*

*While the NAOP is no longer active, the tradition of
International Childfree Day continues. In recent years,
it has gained more recognition through social media and
online communities. Some childfree groups organize local
meetups or online events to mark the day.*

REASON #1

I'd Rather Pack Suitcases Than Diaper Bags
(Childfree Friend's Story)

As I'm writing this section of the book, I'm currently at a public library in Sitka, Alaska, overlooking Baranof Island. I moved here for a seasonal job, and because I needed to escape the "hustle & bustle" lifestyle I'd become accustomed to in Phoenix, AZ and Atlanta, GA.

The weather in Sitka today is gloomy with intermittent rain, and a high of 50 degrees in early June. (MUCH different from the 100+ degree weather in Phoenix during the summer.) Despite the conditions outside, Sitka, AK is just what I need during this phase of my life. It's a quaint town with roughly 9,000 residents, surrounded by beautiful, scenic mountains, clean, crisp air, and it's very walkable. This is a breath of fresh air for me, and Alaska will forever hold a special place in my heart. Ok, enough. Let's discuss my friend *Jane…

Jane, a spunky and sassy older lady, has been adventurous since the first moment we met. During our first talk in the cafeteria at our old job, she revealed that she once ate a fried cockroach while visiting Thailand. It was a dare from her classmates who traveled abroad with her one semester during her college years. Then, she shared her tradition of parasailing every time she visited a new country. That was her "thing." Sometimes, she'd post her adventures on social media. Other times, Jane chose to simply enjoy life outside of social media. I don't blame her for that.

We remained in contact after leaving our old job, and Jane never expressed her desire to not have children, until recently. Unlike most people, I try to keep my nose out of other people's business - because there are SO many other things to discuss. I had no idea Jane was about that childfree life until she was booking a trip to Iceland, when she proclaimed out of the blue, "Ya know, I'd much rather pack suitcases than diaper bags." *Say whattt!* See, I KNEW we were friends for a reason!

In the most polite and non-intrusive way possible, I asked Jane why she decided to not have children. She said, "I don't really have a "*real*" reason. Motherhood was something I chose not to do with my life. When I was younger, of course I got a lot of pushback, but I told them I'd rather travel and move around freely for the rest of my life." And that was pretty much the end of that conversation. Jane's feelings regarding being childfree are completely valid and understandable. All I could do was nod in agreement. She finished booking her Iceland trip right before clocking out of work that evening. Later that year, I booked a flight to Aruba to celebrate my birthday, solely inspired by Jane.

Takeaway: Being childfree equates freedom. You have the freedom to explore the world or live in different cities/states/countries, if that's what you want to do. Relish in this freedom and enjoy your childfree life, unapologetically.

REASON #2

"Because I Simply Don't Want To!"
(My Advice To You)

Take a moment to reflect on the conversation between myself and the man at the airport in Taipei (Introduction section). Have you ever encountered such an authentic, in depth conversation with a stranger while living in (or visiting) the United States? Not to be a Debby Downer, but chances are…probably not.

Now, reflect on a time when someone asked you one of the Common 3 Questions (*What do you do for a living? How many kids do you have? Are you married or in a relationship?*). When they learned you were childfree and didn't want children, what was their next response? I can almost guarantee they judged you and asked, "*What's wrong with you?"* You probably felt inclined to give an elaborate answer and assure them that you're not a bad person. I know this is true because I'm a reformed people-pleaser. However, you DON'T have to overly explain your childfree choice to anyone.

When someone questions your childfree choice and expects you to give a lengthy response about why you chose not to have children, you can just say, "Because I simply don't want to." PERIOD! That's sufficient. Oftentimes, people who choose not to have children are judged, misunderstood, and ostracized by others. They make us feel like our decision *requires* justification. I'm here to tell you it does not. You are not obligated to provide a detailed explanation about what you choose to do with your own body.

I used to over-explain my reasons for not wanting children. Although I was annoyed, I'd respond with, "I love children, but I never wanted to experience pregnancy." Sometimes, I'd say, "I'm not much of a baby person, and the sound of babies crying annoys me." Needless to say, those responses opened up a whole can of worms that could've been avoided if I would've simply said, "I just don't want children."

Admittedly, I don't mind answering the question, "Do you have children?" However, when people rudely accuse me of being selfish and berate me with questions about **WHY** I don't have them, ummm…Houston, we have a problem. All too often, we feel the need to be defensive toward these kinds of people. Doesn't it always seem to be parents who judge and criticize childfree people? It's important to understand that most times they're jealous and resentful of their own life decisions.

Some people can be very nosey and intrusive too. They don't realize that the decision to not have children can be very personal and multifaceted. It could stem from various reasons; ranging from concerns about overpopulation, prioritizing career aspirations, personal fulfillment, or simply not feeling the desire to parent. Whatever the reason(s) may be, it's deserving of respect and acknowledgement.

Takeaway: Your childfree choice should not be scrutinized nor judged by others. To potentially avoid this from happening, say this to a seemingly judgmental person, "I do not have children because I simply do not want them. End of discussion."

REASON #3

Children Are Expensive.

According to recent data and inflation statistics, it costs $331,933 to raise a child from birth until 18 years old. Daycare also costs $2400/month at some facilities.

I am currently debt-free. Well, actually, my consumer debt is paid off. Student loan debt is a whole 'nother story, but I'm making plans to aggressively pay it off. Also, I'm somewhat of a minimalist that chooses not to spend money on unnecessary things. We both know that children ask for unnecessary things at grocery stores, malls, and pretty much everywhere else, right? Right.

My 3rd reason for not having children is to simply preserve my money. From a newborn to adulthood, my (proverbial) child would obviously need love, time, and attention - but they'd also need adequate funds. My student loans are in the 5-figure range. Why in the *bleep* would I add *more* debt to my life by having a child?!?!

Furthermore, I "drank the Kool-Aid" regarding going to college, getting a "good" job, and buying a car and newly-built townhome. I ended up regretting all of those things. The college degree was nothing more than an expensive piece of paper. The job and unnecessary politics involved with upper management ruined my mental health. Oh, and I got tired of driving everyday too. Then, the nonsensical rules within the Homeowners Association (HOA) made owning a home a living hell for me. Knowing all of this, I understand I'm **not** a conformist…so I'm definitely not buying into the idea of starting a family, simply because it's what I'm *supposed* to do with my life after a certain age. Tuh!

Parents say that having children is a rewarding experience, and I'm not here to negate nor confirm that. It could be very rewarding, but it is also expensive. Things add up even BEFORE a child is born - such as purchasing maternity clothes, the pregnancy photoshoot, converting an extra room into a nursery, etc. Then there's the costs associated with giving birth, buying diapers, clothes, baby food, paying for babysitters…the list goes on.

Budgeting for a child is recommended, but not everyone has the foresight or ability to do so. If I'm being honest, I was in my early 30's when I finally decided to stick to a budget for <u>my own life</u> - let alone someone else's. Even if I were extremely wealthy, I still don't believe I'd have children.

In fact, major costs involving raising children include housing, food, childcare/education, health care, and clothing. A breakdown of these costs, as outlined by Northwestern Mutual revealed the average two-parent household with one child will spend:

29% on housing
18% on food
16% on childcare and education 9% on healthcare
7% on miscellaneous expenses 6% on clothing

All in all, the costs involved with planning for and raising a child are overwhelming for me. I didn't even mention things like saving for college, a wedding, or assisting with a down payment for a house. Whew! When does it stop? Spoiler alert: It DOESN'T!! Parenthood is a lifetime job, darling.

Takeaway: While having children can be rewarding for some, the costs associated with taking care of them outweigh the fulfillment for others. It is perfectly OK to forfeit having a child for the sole reason of having extra money in the bank to travel, invest, donate, take care of nieces/nephews, or whatever else you want to do. Never allow others to make you feel bad for choosing to do what is best for you.

Childfree Fact #2

Did you know Ellen Peck advocated for the childfree community in 1971 through her book, 'The Baby Trap?' It was one of the earliest books to explain that being childfree was a valid option for a woman. During 1971, the word "childfree" wasn't created, therefore, Peck called it being "voluntary childless."

The Price is Right:
Bob Barker's Childfree Story

"A person who has never owned a dog has missed a wonderful part of life."

-Bob Barker
(December 12, 1923 - August 26, 2023)

I remember watching 'The Price is Right' with my grandmother during those mornings she'd babysit me, before I was old enough to go to school. I'll never forget Barker's infectious personality, the way he laughed, and his oh-so-popular phrase, "Come on down, you're the next contestant on The Price is Right!"

Barker's decision to remain childfree was a significant personal choice that defined his life and career. For Barker, this decision aligned with his dedication to his work and his deep passion for animal rights, which became another facet of his identity.

Barker was married to his high school sweetheart, Dorothy Jo Gideon, for 36 years until her death in 1981. The couple, though deeply in love, decided not to have children. Barker rarely spoke in depth about the reasons behind their decision, but he and Dorothy shared a life centered on mutual interests, including their love of animals and commitment to vegetarianism. In interviews, Barker indicated that he and his wife were completely content in their lives together and did not feel the need to have children to complete their happiness. I love this!

The freedom Barker had by not having children allowed him to focus on his demanding career and the causes he was passionate about. For over five decades, Barker captivated audiences with his charm, wit, and smooth hosting style on *The Price Is Right*, becoming a household name. Despite the pressures of fame, Barker remained grounded, and his decision to stay childfree enabled him to fully commit to his professional life without the added responsibility of raising children.

Beyond television, Barker's legacy is strongly linked to his advocacy for animal rights, which became a defining piece of his public life after his wife's passing. He became a fierce advocate for animal welfare, donating millions of dollars to organizations like the Sea Shepherd Conservation Society and founding the DJ&T Foundation, named after his wife and mother, to fund low-cost spaying and neutering clinics. Barker famously ended every episode of *The Price Is Right* with the phrase, "Help control the pet population. Have your pets spayed or neutered," a message that reflected his deep commitment to the cause.

Barker's decision to remain childfree allowed him to focus on these personal passions, leaving behind a legacy that included not only his groundbreaking work in television but also his contributions to animal welfare. His life was a testament to the idea that one can live fully and make an enduring impact without following traditional societal expectations, such as parenthood. Bob Barker's story continues to inspire those who seek to carve their own paths.

REASON #4

It's Not My Obligation to Make Them Grandparents

'll never forget the first time my dad approached me about having children. I believe I was either 18 or 19, and we were on the phone having small talk. At the time, he lived in New Jersey, and I was in Indianapolis, IN, attending college. After receiving some advice from him about dating, he jokingly said, "Don't be in a rush to make me a grandfather." I not-so-jokingly said, "You don't have to worry about that, because I don't ever want children and I'm not having them."

After I told him that I didn't want children, he calmly said, "Ok. That's your decision and your choice. No judgment." After that, I didn't hear anything else from him about being a grandfather. I still think about this conversation we had, and I wish I had the opportunity to thank him for not pressuring me to have a child before he passed away. RIP, Dad. 🕊️ Deep down inside, I knew he probably wanted to experience being a grandparent. Or else, he wouldn't have mentioned it, right? They say there's some element of truth behind each joke.

My mother, on the other hand…whew! It seemed like almost every family gathering I attended resulted in her (and others) wondering when I'd have children - especially as I approached 30 years old. Why do most people act like age 30 is the end all, be all? At age 30, society pressures us to no end and they believe we're supposed to have a stable job by 30, be married, and have *at least* one child.

Some parents may start hinting or openly discussing grandchildren as soon as their child surpasses age 25 or gets married, often disregarding the child's personal timeline or circumstances. While both male and female eldest children can face this pressure, it's often more intense for women due to *biological clock* concerns and traditional gender roles. Luckily, as societal norms evolve, there's growing recognition and acceptance of diverse life choices, including being childfree. This is slowly reducing the pressure in <u>some</u> families and communities.

I vividly remember my mother putting me on the spot in front of family members and co-workers (when I'd visit her job), saying things like, "This is the one who hasn't made me a grandmother yet." Or, "I wish my oldest daughter would make me some grandbabies." I'd either ignore the statements, find a way to change the topic, or secretly wish I'd stay home. Eventually, I made the wise decision to protect my peace and avoided attending family gatherings by staying at home. **Why** didn't I think of that sooner?

The pressure that parents often put on their eldest children to produce grandchildren is very common. This pressure can manifest in various ways and have tremendous impacts on family dynamics and individual well-being. In many cultures, there's an expectation that children, especially the eldest, will continue the family line. However, the reality is that we're not obligated to carry on the lineage and make them grandparents.

Reflection: Think about when your parents first mentioned having grandchildren to you. How did that make you feel? What was your response? What would you tell them if they're still pressuring you about having a child (or multiple children)? Write your thoughts below.

REASON #5

Tokophobia
(Fear of Pregnancy) Is a REAL Thing!

I have an astronomical fear of pregnancy and giving birth, and it's always been this way. Blame it on movies I saw as a young child that featured women in the delivery room giving birth. Although I knew it wasn't real, all of the screaming, panting, sweating, and blood utterly grossed me out! It seemed painful and stressful. Thus, pregnancy was always a huge NO THANKS for me.

Tokophobia, according to Google, is defined as a pathological fear of pregnancy which leads to avoidance of childbirth. It can be best described as a morbid fear of childbirth in a woman, who has no previous experience of pregnancy. Did you know this was a thing? I surely didn't. In fact, I was trying to conjure up the right words to describe my fear of pregnancy and giving birth. Now, I can just say, "I have tokophobia" when people ask me why I choose not to have children.

Pregnancy and childbirth seem both burdensome and painful. The fact that I'd be restricted to sleeping a certain way for weeks at a time, gaining excessive weight, and subjecting myself to (potentially) having morning sickness doesn't appeal to me. I don't like the smell, taste, nor the look of vomit, so I would get repulsed if I were to become pregnant and experience morning sickness.

Then, the birthing process…OMG!!! Thanks to social media, (no seriously, THANK YOU to the mothers who are transparent about childbirth), I've seen all I needed to see. There's absolutely no way I would agree to being in labor for several hours (or days) and have someone tearing away at my insides for the sake of experiencing "unconditional love." There's no guarantee that a child will grow up and love their parents unconditionally *anyway*, but that's another story.

As I further researched tokophobia, it's mentioned that the condition is an anxiety disorder, stemming from traumatic experiences, such as witnessing difficult births in the past. Others may develop tokophobia due to a fear of pain, loss of control, or concerns about the well-being of themselves or their baby (if they're on the fence about having children). Rightfully so, this fear can be debilitating, leading to avoidance of pregnancy or extreme anxiety during prenatal care and childbirth.

Takeaway: Tokophobia is a real thing. You shouldn't feel ashamed nor "weird" if you identify with the symptoms and descriptions of tokophobia.

P.S. I recorded a YouTube video that further explains tokophobia and why this is one of my reasons for being childfree. (Search: Childfree_Jerra & "tokophobia" on YouTube to watch the video.)

REASON #6

Why Age 15 Confirmed My Childfree Choice.

In addition to my grotesque fear of pregnancy and childbirth, being a babysitter at age 15 FURTHER confirmed my childfree choice. I guess we can say my tokophobia, in addition to my babysitting experience at 15 were the two catalysts for my decision to not have children.

Growing up, I was always very mature for my age. As the eldest of three children, I remember a lot of responsibilities being placed on me after we moved from my grandmother's home in Gary, Indiana. That large, brick home housed my grandparents, two uncles, an aunt (occasionally), my mother, stepfather, myself, and two siblings. After I graduated 8th grade, we moved from my grandmother's home to a bi-level across town. Although it was *still* considered Gary, IN, the Miller section was a town that many referred to as the "suburbs" of Gary, IN.

My mother worked 3pm-11pm or midnight (7pm-7am) shifts at the local hospital while my stepfather watched after us when we returned home from school. He worked the day shift at his job, and would already be at home when the school bus dropped us off. However, his definition of "watching" us resulted in him staying in his mancave downstairs, while I cooked for my siblings and cleaned up after them by default. I automatically became a third parent, simply because I was the eldest child.

When I turned 15, I was a sophomore in high school, and many family members started to notice just how organized, studious, and mature I really was for my age. At a family function, I vividly remember being volunteered AND told (volunTOLD) to babysit cousins when their parents were at work or unavailable during the weekends. Did I mention those cousins lived on the same block? Therefore, nearly everyday, I would be entertaining small children after school and on the weekends. I simply wanted to play volleyball after school and attend tournaments on the weekends, instead I was basically forced to be an adult.

The children ranged in ages from 3-10 years old. All of the neediness, whining, crying, and messiness from these children was both overstimulating and overwhelming. I just **knew** when I became an adult, I would not have children. The reason was simply because I wanted to live a peaceful life, void of chaos and a messy environment. The only person I want to clean up after is **myself**. At 15-years-old, I couldn't wait to grow up, move away, and go to college. At least I would finally be responsible for myself and experience solitude for once.

When I mentioned I didn't want children to some family members (I believe I was 17 at the time), I received major backlash. One adult accused me of being pitiful. Others would either dismiss me or say things like, "*You'll change your mind one day,*" or "*We'll see.*" Welp, I guess they SEE now, don't they?! It's crazy how some people think that just because you're young, you don't know what you want (or don't want) out of life.

In hindsight, I'm thankful that I had the experience of babysitting at such a young age. It showed me what my triggers were in terms of overstimulation and sensory overload. 'Till this day, I thrive in solitude, organization, and non-chaotic environments. When I'm around a lot of noise and chaos, I either get an attitude or leave the environment ASAP. I'm pretty sure that if I were to become a parent, I'd resent motherhood during the newborn-toddler phase, because of the crying and whining that ensues. For these reasons, I don't want to/ don't need to have children. I knew what was best for me years ago.

Takeaway: If you're an eldest daughter or son, I empathize with you. I know what it's like to be ladened with adult responsibilities while you're a child. If this is your reason for choosing to be childfree, it's completely valid.

Betty White: A Childfree Icon

"It was a very conscious decision on my part not to have children - which I have never regretted."
- Betty White
(January 17, 1922 - December 31, 2021)

Some people believe that older women will one day regret not having children. However, that's not the case for Betty White (and many others, celebrity or non-celebrity). Betty White's legacy as an actress, comedian, and humanitarian extends beyond her numerous accolades and awards. One of the most notable aspects of her life was her decision to remain childfree, a choice she made with great thought and conviction. White was known for her deep love of animals, her groundbreaking roles in television, and her sharp wit. Yet, her personal decision not to have children also stood out, especially in an era when motherhood was often considered an essential part of a woman's life.

White married three times, and her longest and most cherished marriage was with Allen Ludden, a TV host and personality. Though the two were deeply in love, Betty White made the conscious choice not to have children of her own. In interviews, she spoke openly about her decision, expressing no regrets. White was candid, saying that while she loved children, her focus on her career and other passions made her feel that motherhood wasn't the right path for her. Her transparency about this decision was refreshing, especially given the societal expectations of women during much of her lifetime.

Betty White's decision to remain childfree allowed her to pursue her many interests with dedication. She often credited this choice as part of the reason she could devote so much time to her career and her advocacy for animal welfare. White was a lifelong advocate for animals, working with organizations such as the Los Angeles Zoo and the Morris Animal Foundation. She used her platform to champion causes close to her heart, believing that her time and energy could be better spent on these endeavors. For her, being childfree provided the freedom to focus on making a difference in the lives of animals and people alike.

Her legacy is also notable in how it normalized the idea that a woman could have a fulfilling, impactful life without children. White did not see her choice as a lack or something missing; rather, it was a personal decision that fit with her goals, values, and passions. This perspective resonated with many people, especially women who felt pressured by societal expectations to have children. White's openness about her life choices helped to broaden the narrative about what it means to live a full and meaningful life.

All in all, Betty White's life was a testament to living authentically and embracing one's own path. Her decision to remain childfree did not define her, but it was an integral part of how she approached her own life. She demonstrated that a person could create an enduring legacy of love, laughter, and compassion in countless ways. Her story continues to inspire generations to pursue their passions, live on their terms, and embrace the choices that bring them fulfillment.

REASON #7

I Choose to Birth IDEAS, Not Babies.

At a very young age, I noticed I was different. While other girls were desiring the attention of boys at the playground, I was sitting with the teacher, reading during recess. My mind was always on creating, writing, and *being in my own little world.* As I grew older, the desire to create and innovate only intensified. I was never interested in motherhood because I knew it would slow down or potentially halt my creative endeavors. Yes…I understand there are mothers who still create and own businesses, and I commend them for that. I really do. However, that doesn't mean I need to follow their path in life.

In my 20s, as friends and high school classmates started having families, I dove headfirst in my career. I was blessed enough to work at a municipal government job in accounting, then was promoted to Payroll Manager. Although the job wasn't something I wanted to do long-term, I was grateful for a steady paycheck. That paycheck helped fund my first book (that's now out-of-print). *This is an entire story for another day…but because of the shady experience with the publisher of my first book, I now choose to self-publish, instead of trusting someone else to publish for me.* OK, moving right along…

Late-night brainstorming sessions, followed by early meetings at work, and the "grind" fueled my days. I loved seeing my ideas come to life - whether they were baking/decorating cakes, writing blogs, or revising resumes and doing career coaching. Each successful venture felt like a birth - a creation I nurtured and watched grow into something impactful and meaningful.

I fully understand the world is full of ways to nurture, care, and create, and they don't involve parenthood. During the pandemic, I learned how to care for plants. Many years ago, I also learned how to self-publish books and helped others write and self-publish their books too. Each of these endeavors was comparable to planting a seed and watching it bloom, offering a sense of purpose and connection that was extremely fulfilling. My ideas being cultivated into products and gifts for others to consume is rewarding enough for me. I don't need to push a baby out of my vuh-jay in order to be fulfilled in life. When parents tell me their children bring them fulfillment, I understand where they're coming from - but it doesn't influence me to change my mind about my childfree choice.

As mentioned previously, the choice to remain childfree was hardly understood or accepted by those around me. Family gatherings often included subtle (and not so subtle) hints about the *joys of motherhood*. They didn't seem to understand/care that I find joy in mentoring youth (I was a substitute teacher and HigherEd professional in my 30's), volunteering for causes I believe in, and dedicating myself to projects that make a difference.

Takeaway: Understand there is <u>no</u> one way to seek purpose in life. Some may find fulfillment in parenthood, and that's totally fine. Life is all about doing what's best for YOU, and if you discover birthing ideas - instead of babies is most fulfilling, that's 100% valid.

REASON #8

I Don't Care About Being Fruitful & Multiplying.

If you also experienced a religious upbringing, then you have probably heard about the "*Be fruitful and multiply*" scripture that's been ingrained in us. This scripture came from Genesis 1:8, where God instructs us to "*Be fruitful and multiply and fill the Earth*." When God speaks of being fruitful and multiplying, He is speaking about procreation of the human species.

This scripture <u>AND</u> Genesis (The Bible chapter) were written in the Old Testament - a time when the earth NEEDED to be replenished! Currently, we have over 8 billion people on the planet. There's certainly no need to replenish this overpopulated world right now…we have enough people. As they often say in Atlanta, Georgia, "WE FULL!"

Quite frequently, when women speak up about not having children - especially in Christian communities, they're met with disdain, dismissal, and disappointments. Aren't Christians supposed to be loving members of society that shouldn't judge others' decisions? Hmph. Sounds like a lot of hypocrisy to me. As long as someone's life decisions aren't associated with theft, violence, laziness, lying, or murder, I have no opinion or judgment whatsoever.

I can recall various YouTube subscribers who have reached out to me from the Christian community, to express how they were outcast by church members simply because they chose to not have children. Based on what they experienced, I can understand why some women feel the need to be silent about their childfree choice. I was that way for several years, until I discovered the confidence and IDGAF-ness to speak up about being childfree. It's crazy how the opinions of others will shame some people into silence. It should be the other way around though - judgmental people ought to feel the urge to be quiet about a person's desire to remain childfree.

The archaic belief that we *still* need to be fruitful and multiply in this day and age is nonsensical. Again, there are enough people in this world and some areas are severely overpopulated. Also, why is being fruitful and multiplying *solely* associated with having children??? Being fruitful and multiplying can also mean being productive and achieving growth in different areas, such as personal development, career advancement, or community contributions. It involves creating positive outcomes, increasing your impact, and continuously developing new skills and opportunities.

Takeaway: You can still honor God and remain childfree. Being fruitful and multiplying means so much more than just having children. You shouldn't feel ashamed nor silenced for your childfree choice, so proclaim it **UNAPOLOGETICALLY**. You're still a good and honorable person.

Childfree Fact #3

Did you know Jesus was **unmarried** and **childfree**? It's true. There's no evidence in The Bible that indicates He had children or was married. Yet, Jesus was still able to live a fruitful life and accomplish great things.

The next time someone reminds you of God's word to "Be fruitful and multiply," tell them Jesus didn't have children, and watch their reaction. ☺

REASON #9

I'd Rather Be An Aunt.

I was 30 years old when my nephew was born - the age when society constantly reminded me that my "biological clock" was ticking. This was also the age when I thought I had to have everything *figured out* in life. I was (and still am) unmarried with no children. Although I lived alone in my apartment, I didn't have a home of my own at age 30. I also had a dead-end job that I despised. Needless to say, I felt like a complete failure on the inside. Then, my sister revealed she was pregnant. While congratulating her, I quietly said to myself, "*Whoo-hoo!*" because I knew my mother would finally stop pressuring ME (the eldest sibling) to give her a grandchild.

You probably won't believe this, but there was a time when I *thought* I wanted to have a child one day. I was involved in a serious relationship, and somehow I felt having his baby was the next step that would solidify our bond. Plus, a lot of people (including my ex-boyfriend) told me I'd make a great mother. I had to take a step back and really dig deep to understand those were nothing but societal expectations trying to convince me to change my mind about having children. I honestly can't picture myself taking care of a baby nor toddler 24/7 - it would drive me crazy! Obviously, I'm SO grateful that I came to my senses and never had children.

I must say that being an aunt to my amazing nephew, Cameron, is great for me. He's such a joy to be around, but when I need my alone time, I revel in the fact that I can take him right back to my sister's house. That's an amazing feeling. I'm part of the village that helps to take care of him. I cherish our bond and the fact that I can witness Cameron's growth and development without the full-time responsibilities and commitment of parenthood.

I have the privilege of being his confidante, mentor, and future international travel buddy. We share a secret handshake, inside jokes, and love for the great outdoors. Being his aunt means that I spoil him with gifts and his favorite sour candies, plan fun outings and adventures, and build lasting connections without the day-to-day demands of being a parent. Even if I had to be Cameron's sole caretaker, that would be a job I'd take great pride in, because he's such an awesome kid.

<blockquote>
Takeaway: Parenthood isn't for everyone, and that's OK. Continue to love on your niece(s) and/or nephew(s) and make lifelong memories. Enjoy spending time with yourself and loved ones, if you're not an aunt/uncle.
</blockquote>

REASON #10

Legacy and Pregnancy are NOT Interrelated!

It's very interesting how some people confuse legacy with lineage, and assume that creating a family is the only way to achieve legacy. Contrary to popular belief, it **IS** possible to still have a legacy while being childfree. Legacy is defined as "the long-lasting impact of particular events, actions, etc. that took place in the past, or of a person's life." Clearly, the definition of legacy doesn't mention being a parent. Many people misunderstand the meaning of this word.

Lineage, on the other hand, is associated with one's ancestors. It involves the preceding members of a person's family, who are directly related to that person. Based on these breakdowns, I believe LINEAGE is the word people

<u>should</u> use when they assume childfree people won't have a legacy.

Furthermore, the deliberate choice to not have children doesn't imply that childfree people will lead non-fulfilling lives, and won't have a legacy. Legacy is established through various acts - such as charitable giving, developing close friendships, or even your sense of style. How do people describe you when you're not in the room? What do people mostly know you for? How would you like to be remembered? The answers to these questions signify your legacy, or in other words, the impact you leave on others.

I know a childfree person that owns a business and employs teenagers and young adults. After hours, the business owner also mentors youth in the community and teaches them about entrepreneurship. Although this person doesn't have children of their own, they're still making a positive impact on others lives - essentially building a legacy.

Another way to build legacy is through acts of kindness and generosity. Giving someone a compliment, allowing people to merge over into traffic (instead of speeding up like a maniac), or doing volunteer work are all profound. The positive impact on communities and individuals from acts of kindness and generosity are impactful and everlasting - which is essentially part of your legacy.

Takeaway: The essence of legacy is the lasting difference one makes in the world. For example, people associate Steve Jobs with Apple. I literally had to research how many children he had. His four children have nothing to do with his legacy, but Apple does. Catch my drift?

P.S. I did a virtual presentation on this topic at the Childless Collective Summit in 2023. The title was 'Legacy and Pregnancy are NOT Interrelated.' I uploaded the video on my YouTube channel, @Childfree_Jerra.

REASON #11

Children are TOO NOISY!

There's a reel on Instagram that's been making its rounds. The audio involves loud, shrieking crying from a baby. I had to mute the sound in order to enjoy reading the captions and comments from others on IG. If the video itself is bothersome to me…I can only imagine if I were a parent, having to deal with that noise everyday in real life. Yikes!

In fact, I'm writing this chapter while sitting in a somewhat busy coffee shop. Sometimes, I need to step away from my home office in order to garner inspiration and spark creativity. This particular establishment is the perfect environment - with its caramel-colored walls, warm, cozy fireplace, amidst oversized dark brown microfiber chairs. The sound of jazz music playing in the background and heavy rain outside is drowned out by a whiny toddler who appears to be cranky about something. She keeps throwing bread on the floor and making pouty faces, while exclaiming, "I wanna go home!" *Honey, I wish you'd take your a** home too!* I wish I could say that out loud LOL.

If I had to deal with this type of behavior everyday, my mental health would deteriorate. Studies have shown that prolonged exposure to loud, unpredictable, and uncontrollable sounds can affect one's well being. For example, it can increase stress levels, interfere with sleep patterns, and even contribute to anxiety and depression. Because I deeply value peace and quiet, dealing with the noise and chaos from a baby/toddler would be very challenging for me.

Granted, I'm in a public place and it's unfair of me to expect that there wouldn't be at least *some* type of noise, the temper tantrum this child is throwing is a bit much. I'm wearing headphones too, but since I know the baby is here, I'm still affected. The parents seem to be unphased by her behavior. (Why are some parents like this?) It's almost like they have blinders on, regarding her behavior. When my nephew was younger, thankfully, he didn't embarrass us in public…which leads me to believe that some parents probably don't set expectations with children prior to leaving the home.

Although the noise from babies and toddlers is a lot, children tend to make noise as they grow older too. Imagine a school-aged child taking up drumming, or learning how to play the flute after school. Or, constantly arguing with siblings and playing video games loudly. Then, there are (some) teenagers who enjoy blasting music loudly throughout the house. This constant auditory stimulation can be overwhelming, especially for those like myself, who thrive in tranquil environments.

Clearly, the need for quiet time for work or personal activities is increasingly difficult to achieve with children in the home. As a writer, having peace and quiet are essential to my effectiveness and quality of writing. That said, it's time for me to leave this coffee shop and go home - the noise from this child is unbearable.

Takeaway: If you notice your mood changing when you hear children crying or making any type of sudden noise, it is perfectly normal. There is nothing wrong with you if you prefer serene environments. From infancy to teenage years, children can disrupt your peace and quiet, and it's OK if you choose not to have them solely for this reason.

Childfree Fact #4

Did you know George Washingtion, the first President of the United States was childfree? While he did not have biological children of his own, Washington was a devoted stepfather.

He married Martha Custis in 1759, who was a widow with two children from her previous marriage. Washington helped raise and care for Martha's children, John Parke Custis (known as "Jacky") and Martha Parke Custis (known as "Patsy"), but George Washington never had children of his own.

REASON #12

I'm Too Selfish With My Time

People who criticize the childfree lifestyle refere to us as selfish. Huh??? Selfish toward WHOM, exactly? Our unborn child(ren)? Make it make sense. How can we be selfish toward someone that doesn't even exist? I think it's actually selfish and irresponsible for a parent to have a child knowing good and well they can't properly provide for them.

Also, there's nothing wrong with being labeled as selfish. In this life, we *have* to be selfish to an extent and preserve certain parts of ourselves, in order to function. That said, embrace your selfishness and disregard those who view it as a bad thing.

I believe time is of the essence, and I simply don't have the time to potty train someone, teach them alphabets & numbers, or take care of them 24/7. I have my own dreams to chase, passions to pursue, and flights to catch. Yes, yes…I know there are people who do these things while raising children, but I simply choose not to. The more uninterrupted, quiet time I have, the better my mental state is.

Aside from working and making a living, I'd rather spend my free time reading self-improvement books, listening to podcasts, hiking, and traveling. I don't have time (nor am I interested in creating time) to sing lullabies, wipe diapers, or breastfeed.

In a nutshell, being childfree equates to having freedom. That freedom creates abundant time to do whatever we choose to do. Having children is a huge responsibility, and honestly, I commend those who have taken time to consider all factors, and STILL choose to be parents anyway.

We're living in a world where time is our most precious commodity. It is a 100% valid choice to not have children because of the time it takes to raise them properly. Let people say what they want, but at least you know you're making a decision that makes sense for you. You're allowed to be selfish with your time and there's nothing wrong with that.

Reflection:

Write down 5 things that you have adequate time to do, simply because you're childfree. These things can involve having more time to sleep in, traveling, working on your car/home, etc.

Rosa Parks Was Childfree Too

"I would like to be remembered as a person who wanted to be free…so other people would also be free."

- Rosa Parks, Civil Rights Activist
(February 4, 1913 - October 24, 2005)

Did you know that Rosa Parks didn't have children? If you didn't know, don't feel bad. Most people aren't aware of this important fact either. When I first mentioned that Rosa Parks was childfree on my Instagram page, many were enlightened and surprised.

Aside from Corretta Scott King, and many others, Rosa Parks was one of the most recognized women during the Civil Rights era in America. She was born in 1913 in Tuskegee, Alabama and later moved to Montgomery, Alabama to attend school. Her mother was a teacher and instilled the value of education in Rosa Parks at a very young age.

Parks had siblings, but one can assume she was probably the eldest child. I say this because she delayed finishing school until 20 years old to be a caretaker of her mother and grandmother. When she finally finished school in the 1930's, she was amongst 6% of other Black students who also graduated during that time. Rosa Parks' husband encouraged her to finish her high school education after they got married.

Parks is best known for refusing to give up a seat to a white man on a segregated bus in Montgomery, Alabama. Her actions led her to become a courageous and unapologetic leader of the bus boycott, which lasted 381 days. After the boycott ended, Rosa and her husband were harassed, became unemployed, and received threats to leave Montgomery. As a result, they relocated to Detroit.

Rosa Parks and her husband, Raymond Parks, never had children. They were married from 1932 until his death in 1977, but the couple never had children of their own. While she did not have children, Parks was very involved in youth activism and education. She often worked with young people in civil rights organizations and gave talks at schools to inspire new generations to continue the fight for equality.

Rosa Parks' childfree status wasn't widely discussed during her lifetime, as it wasn't considered particularly relevant to her civil rights work. However, it's an interesting aspect of her personal life that deserves attention.

Some key points about Rosa Parks' childfree status:

- **Choice vs. Circumstance**: It's not entirely clear whether Parks and her husband Raymond chose not to have children or if they were unable to conceive. This ambiguity is common for many historical figures, as infertility and reproductive choices were often not openly discussed.

- **Focus on Activism**: Not having children may have allowed Parks to dedicate more time and energy to her civil rights work. Her activism often required long hours, travel, and sometimes put her in dangerous situations.
- **Mentorship Role**: Though she didn't have biological children, Parks took on a mentorship role for many young activists. She was particularly involved with youth programs in the NAACP and other civil rights organizations.
- **Historical Context**: In the early to mid-20th century, being childfree was less common and often more stigmatized than it is today. However, Parks' prominent role in the civil rights movement likely overshadowed any societal pressure she might have faced regarding her childfree status.
- **Legacy**: Despite not having descendants, Parks left a lasting legacy through her activism and the inspiration she provided to generations of civil rights advocates.

REASON #13

Young, Married, & Childfree: Clarence & Janet's (Childfree Friend's) Story

I met *Clarence* and *Janet,* a young, black, intelligent, and thriving couple at a real estate conference a few years ago. Their welcoming energy instantly drew me in, and I quickly realized we had a lot in common - especially in terms of being childfree.

We didn't get a chance to speak much during the conference, but they invited me to dinner at a nearby restaurant after the conference. Being the somewhat picky and lactose intolerant person I am, I ordered a "safe" meal that didn't contain dairy, and it didn't disappoint! Janet ordered lasagna and salad, while Clarence ordered a steak with mashed potatoes and asparagus.

While we waited on our entrees, we had small talk about our careers, life in general, and you guessed it… being childfree! Clarence described how he knew since age 4 that he didn't want children (more on that story later). I burst out laughing when he compared holding a baby to picking up a cat! LOL! Now that I think about it, it's *definitely* similar! The vertebrae and "wiggly-ness" of a baby compared to a feline is hilarious, yet oh so true!

Janet told me she was on the fence about having children. She loves them, but also understands parenthood is a 24/7, year-round job that doesn't stop when a child turns 18 - it's a lifelong commitment. "What if I end up raising someone that still needs help in their 40's & 50's?", she says. Extremely valid point. That's something I believe most people don't take into consideration before having children.

Janet was raised in a two-parent, Jamaican household in the suburbs of New York. She had a great childhood that can be compared to the Huxtables, except she only has one younger sister. Janet was raised in a traditional home, however her parents never pressured her nor her sister to have children. Her dad simply wanted (and still wants) the best for his daughters. Mom, on the other hand has expressed that she would love to have grandchildren, but has recently accepted it may never happen, and she's OK with that. Janet's younger sister is pretty headstrong and adamant about not having children.

Clarence, the youngest sibling, was raised in Providence, Rhode Island and spent a vast majority of his childhood with a babysitter. This babysitter also watched several other children, and Clarence noticed how manipulative, unruly, and problematic some children are. I'm probably telling my age here, but remember the *Rugrats* cartoon? Yeah…that's how he best describes those children. "They kept pretending to be hurt, were always finessing the babysitter, and they were just downright mean! That's when I realized I didn't like children," Clarence says. Mind you, he was just FOUR YEARS OLD when he came to this realization. Also, Clarence's older sister had children young, and he helped raise them - ages 2, 4, & 8. "In my mind, I *already* had kids," he mentions.

When Clarence and Janet were still dating, they went to one of Janet's family functions. One of her uncles said to Clarence, "You'd make a good dad." Clarence was always transparent and forthcoming with Janet about his desire to not have children, so you can probably imagine how uncomfortable this made him feel.

At another family gathering, Janet's grandfather asked them, "When are you gonna have some kids?" They had only been married for a year. ONE WHOLE YEAR. The grandfather continued probing, then said to Clarence in a very condescending tone, "What's the matter? *Don't you know how to **do it**?*" Yikes! On the other hand, Clarence's family never asked nor pressured him about having children. They simply accepted his life decision and stayed in their own lane.

Let's get into the deeper reasons why this couple is postponing and/or choosing not to have children. Clarence and Janet shared certain conversations they have with co-workers and how their lives seem so hectic outside of work. Those co-workers frequently talked about attending soccer games on the weekends, helping with homework during the week, going to school plays, etc., while Clarence and Janet listened - silently thanking God they're not in that predicament.

Then, Clarence went into detail about the broken educational system. "I thought school didn't make sense when I was in kindergarten!," he says. He also mentioned how schools keep children away from home for 7-8 hours, essentially taking the place of their parent(s), while "teaching" them a copy/paste system that has proven to be ineffective. "The whole robotic way of doing things… go to school, graduate, go to college, get in debt, get a job, work for 30-40 years, then finally retire…has been ingrained in people's minds for several years - and it all starts with the broken school system. Why would I want to raise a child in this mess? If (and that's a **STRONG** "if") I want to have children, they would definitely be homeschooled."

Also, Janet brought to my attention a 2021 CNBC News study which reveals that parents experience a "happiness bump" right after a baby is born. However, that happiness dissolves after a year, as mentioned in the article. Some agree that having children helps to enhance their life experience, but very few are transparent about the amount of responsibility and daily stress/worry it brings. Life can be stressful enough on its own. No need to add children to the equation.

Takeaway: Just because you're married doesn't mean you're *supposed* to have children. The desire to want to have children MUST be there, and it requires thoughtful consideration if you're on the fence. Choosing not to have children doesn't make you selfish - it makes you SELF-AWARE. Lastly, if you change your mind about having children, that's OK. No judgment here.

Childfree Fact #5:

Many people misconstrue the words 'childless' and 'childfree.' Being childfree signifies that you don't have the desire to have children at all. When someone is childless, they may desire children, but are physically unable to have them.

REASON #14

I'm 63, Childfree, & I Have NO Regrets! (Childfree Friend's Story)

Meet Sharon*, an avid traveler, golf aficionado, and a baking enthusiast. She's also a retired government worker who lives in a 3-bedroom home in Arizona. With all of these titles she holds, you BETTER NOT call her granny!

Sharon has known since the age of 23 that she didn't want children. The first time she mentioned this to family, the backlash and insults were so severe that she stopped talking about it for several years. (I can relate to this!)

Growing up, Sharon was the youngest of four children. Her parents were married for 14 years, until her father passed away when she was 10 years old. Growing up, her childhood was fun and bright. Dad worked as a middle manager at a factory, and worked the traditional 8am-4pm shift. Mom stayed at home to take care of household responsibilities and the children. When dad came home during the week, dinner was already prepared. Baked chicken, mashed potatoes, and peas - with 2 slices of garlic toast were dad's favorite. Sharon describes the delightful smile on his face when he'd arrive home. It was a genuine smile, and it seemed like nothing upset dad. "He was always so jovial and easygoing," Sharon describes.

Little did she know, her dad was a functional alcoholic. He and Sharon's mom would get into heated arguments about his drinking very often. No one knew about his bad habit until many years after he passed, because arguments always occurred when children were sleeping upstairs.

When dad passed, life took a 180-degree turn. Mom was no longer taking care of the house, and "meals" consisted of cereal, peanut butter & jelly sandwiches, and pizza that older siblings ordered. Mom grieved for several years and struggled to take care of herself. Sharon observed how older siblings had to take on the role of a parent, while empathizing with her mom.

You might be wondering, *Why did she decide at age 23 to not have children?* Here, I'll tell you…It's because she got involved with a man and discovered he had a drinking problem. She refused to allow history to repeat itself. Rather than sweeping this issue under the rug, she broke up with him. Luckily, they weren't married, which made it easier for her to leave.

Age 23 was the defining number for Sharon, even though her first life-altering event happened at age 10. She vowed to never take dating seriously, frowned upon the idea of marriage, and DEFINITELY chose to be childfree. The uncertainty of having a two-parent household was always in the back of her mind, because she saw firsthand how difficult it was to raise children alone.

Now, at age 63, she's been on countless dates with men, has never been married, and has no children of her own. Sharon is a proud aunt of 2 nephews and 4 nieces, and has a pet German Shepard. In her spare time (which she has PLENTY of), she enjoys baking cookies and muffins for her nieces and nephews, traveling to exotic countries, and playing golf.

She says being childfree is the best life decision she's made, and wouldn't change it for the world. Absolutely NO regrets! "When people told me I'd regret not having children when I was younger, I wish they could see me now!," she says while smiling widely. Aside from activities mentioned earlier, she has also fostered a 60+ community within her neighborhood and they regularly check on each other. Sharon considers them her family, although she has close relationships with her blood family members. This goes to show that family ISN'T exclusive to those who have children, and/or a husband/wife.

Although Sharon is at an age where many of her classmates are grandparents, that's a title that she doesn't hold - and she's proud of it. "The only grands I want in my possession are Grands biscuits," she says jokingly - yet seriously.

Takeaway: When someone tries to shame you for not wanting to have children, remind them that you know what's best for you. Almost everyone has regrets in life, but it's better to regret not having children, than to have them and regret being a parent.

REASON #15

Pregnancy Complications & Death

For some, the decision to remain childfree is directly linked to health concerns. The more I began to research the implications and risks of childbirth and pregnancy, it further confirmed that being childfree is what's best for me. I learned that recent studies reveal that Black women are 3 times more likely to die from pregnancy-related complications than their white counterparts. Also, we (Black women) are more likely to experience life-threatening conditions like preeclampsia, postpartum hemorrhage, and blood clots, as a result of having children.

Those that know me can agree that I tend to be more optimistic about things that happen in life. However, knowing what I know about pregnancy and childbirth - especially in the Black community, I simply cannot turn a blind eye. I don't want to take a chance at losing my own life to give birth to a child.

A Harvard study conducted by Ana Langer stated, "A big reason for the disparity may be racism." Basically, Black women are undervalued. They are not monitored as carefully as white women are. When they do present hospital staff with symptoms, they are often dismissed."

SMH. Reading this truly disgusted me, although I was initially aware of this. The Harvard study then mentioned tennis star, Serena Williams' experience while giving birth. She gave birth to her daughter via cesarean section, and voiced concerns of pain thereafter. As you can probably guess, her concerns were ignored, which resulted in Serena experiencing a pulmonary embolism. All of this could have been avoided if certain medical professionals weren't racist and treated her fairly.

Pregnancy complications are a significant concern for many individuals considering parenthood. These can range from relatively minor issues to life-threatening conditions that put both the mother and child at risk. Some women face increased risks due to pre-existing health conditions, while others may develop complications during pregnancy itself. The potential for these sorts of complications can result in anxiety and fear, greatly influencing the childfree choice. This is an extremely valid and legitimate concern.

It's important to recognize the mental health toll of nearly dying during childbirth that some women experience. It doesn't only occur with Black women, however. Other races have traumatic experiences within and outside the birthing room, including miscarriages, gestational diabetes, and premature babies, to name a few.

Takeaway: While it isn't my intention to paint a bleak picture of childbirth, I do aim to educate you on the risks (especially if you're on the fence about having children). The concern and fear of pregnancy complications that could lead to death are extremely wise reasons to remain childfree.

Arielle's Childfree Story

Arielle is a valuable supporter on my Instagram and YouTube accounts. I reached out to her and asked if she'd be willing to share her childfree story. Thankfully, she obliged. Here's her story:

I didn't realize it at the time, but I believe I made the decision to be childfree at the age of 17. As the eldest of my mother's five children, I spent much of my childhood helping to raise my younger siblings after our father abandoned us. I babysat, cooked meals, changed diapers, helped with homework, and often faced punishment if I couldn't assist or if I dared to pursue my own interests. The only time I ever showed disrespect to a teacher was in high school when she began giving me zeros for arriving late - a situation entirely beyond my control. My mother worked the night shift, leaving me responsible for waking up my siblings, getting them dressed, and either driving them to school before heading to my own or waiting for my mother to return home to take them. In fact, the only reason I was supported in getting a car was so I could transport my siblings or run errands for the family.

At 17, everything came to a head. One day, while I was at school, a social worker pulled me aside to inform me that my mother had been admitted to a mental hospital, and my siblings were being split up and placed into foster care. I cannot begin to express the dehumanizing nature of this experience for all of us. No one who knew us wanted to take us in, so we were forced into the care of people who viewed us as nothing more than a source of income.

During a court hearing where everyone was arguing over who should be forced to take custody, my mother's friend reminded me that in just a few months, I would turn 18 and could take legal guardianship of my siblings. When I told her that I was going to college, she snapped at me, insisting that I wouldn't get to go and that I needed to apply for food stamps and public housing to care for my siblings. My world stopped. At that moment, I realized that I did not want the burden of children. I didn't want to sacrifice my life for my siblings anymore, and I certainly didn't want to have children of my own who would require me to sacrifice myself for them.

Fortunately, my mother's friend was wrong and I was able to attend college out-of-state. For the first time in my life, I was away from my family, free to live for myself, make my own choices, and simply enjoy the freedom of independence. I was finally able to see myself as more than just a tool for others' needs. With this newfound sense of freedom, I knew that I couldn't exist in a household where I had to care for children.

As the years went on and I entered romantic relationships, I was constantly made to feel that I should want children, despite expressing that I didn't have the desire. Many of the women around me were either having children or desperately trying to find a man to have children with. It seemed that a lot of women thought about motherhood in the abstract, without considering the day-to-day realities of raising a child. Having been so involved in raising my siblings, I understood the daily cost of motherhood, and to me, that cost is far too high. I know I would love any child I brought into this world, but I also know myself well enough to understand that I would resent having to be a mother every single day. To me, it wouldn't be fair for a child to grow up with a mother who doesn't truly want to be one.

Beyond the day-to-day responsibilities of motherhood, I also take issue with the reproductive process itself. This might sound silly to some, but I don't think it's fair that men reproduce through an orgasm, while women endure pregnancy - a life-threatening condition - followed by major surgery to give birth. Women go through rough physical, emotional, and hormonal changes, while men face no physical consequences. For women, it's a painful, life-altering experience but it is completely optional. I know I can't change biology, but I'm fortunate enough to have the choice not to participate in it. Many of our ancestors did not have this choice and I think they'd be proud that I am exercising my privilege to make a choice based on my own needs and desires.

After giving birth, society expects women to be the default parents, taking on the majority of the parenting responsibilities, often with little to no support from a partner or people outside of the home. Fatherhood is almost treated as optional or a hobby, yet we all get our fathers' last names. It doesn't really seem balanced to me because women do most of the labor.

The rebellious, anti-capitalist in me views withholding reproduction as an act of resistance. Our society consistently fails to care for its people properly. We lack adequate healthcare, food security, housing, education, and so much more. We are wage slaves for most of our lives, paying taxes, yet we don't receive the care we need in return. Even in the context of childbirth, our country refuses to provide proper maternity leave for women, forcing many to return to work shortly after giving birth because they can't afford to stay home. I don't find these conditions to be suitable for reproduction or raising children.

I have complete peace about my decision to be childfree. It's a choice that has allowed me to craft a life that aligns perfectly with my values and desires. My days are filled with the freedom to pursue my passions, nurture my relationships, and live authentically on my terms. I know without a doubt that I will never regret this decision because it was made with careful thought and complete self-awareness. I understood from an early age that this was the right path for me, and I'm grateful that I had the clarity and courage to choose it.

Thoughts for Other Childfree Women

Choosing to be childfree is a deeply personal decision, and it is one that is entirely valid. Society often pressures women to see motherhood as the ultimate goal, as if our worth is tied to our ability to bear and raise children. But the truth is, your worth is inherent, and your life's purpose is yours to define.

You may have made this choice after reflecting on your experiences. Perhaps you value your independence, your peace, or the freedom to live life on your own terms. Maybe, like many of us, you see the challenges of motherhood and recognize that it's not a lifestyle you wish to embrace. Or perhaps you understand that the societal, physical, and emotional demands placed on mothers are inequitable and unfair, and you have chosen to step away from that expectation.

Whatever your reasons, know they are valid. The decision to live childfree is as legitimate as the decision to become a parent. It's about knowing what's right for you and embracing the lifestyle that brings you fulfillment.

You are not alone in this decision. There are many women who have chosen this path and live happy, meaningful lives. Your choice is a powerful expression of your autonomy and self-awareness. It is a reflection of your understanding of who you are and what you want from life. And that is a beautiful thing.

*Arielle and her content can be found on **YouTube** and **Instagram** @ibuymyownroses.

Acknowledgements

First and foremost, I want to thank God - the divine spirit that resides inside of me. I'm thankful for my gift of writing, creativity, and the ability to live an authentic, fulfilled life.

I'm also grateful for having family members that believe in me. Thank you for affirming me and trusting me to make the right decisions with my life.

To my nephew & proofreader, Cameron, thank you for being a wonderful beacon of light. I foresee a bright future for you, and it's been a joy and pleasure watching you grow up thus far.

To my amazing book cover designers, Monica and Unique, you are truly gifted. Thank you for everything.

Thank you to Holly Meyer, General Manager at Aspen Suites Hotel in Sitka, Alaska. I needed this solitude and serene environment to work on this project. Thank you for hiring me for the Summer 2024 season.

Thank you to the staff at Sitka Public Library. I appreciate your kindness and professionalism. I also appreciate you for allowing me to use the private study room (at late notice) to work on my book with no distractions.

Last, but certainly not least, thank you to my Instagram, YouTube, and TikTok family. I call you my family because we share a common interest on this childfree journey and we deeply understand each other. Your endless support means more to me than you'll ever know.

About The Author

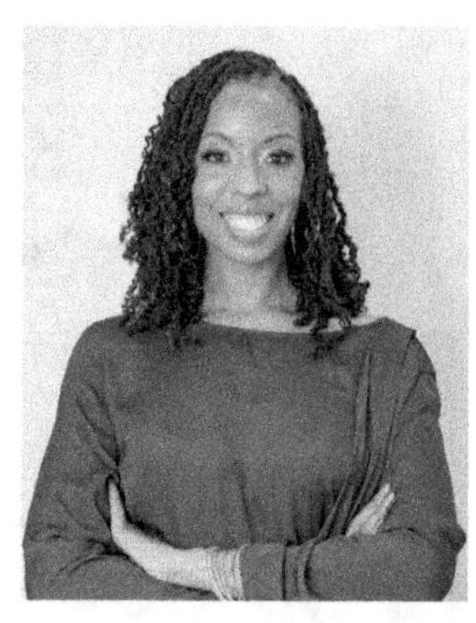

Jerra Latrice Mitchell is an award-winning writer and author. She has authored 4 books to date (2 are out-of-print), and 'I Was Bitter, Now I'm Better' is her first self-published and most treasured book. It is available on Amazon.

In 2021, Jerra founded Unfertilized Eggs®, whose mission was to validate and normalize the childfree community. The company was closed in 2024, and transformed into a personal brand (Childfree Jerra). Jerra now operates her YouTube channel, @Childfree_Jerra under the same pretenses - to validate and normalize the childfree community.

Jerra has been featured in Glamour, Black Women's Expo, Essence Festival, and has spoken on a panel of childfree women at Reddit. Jerra is currently enjoying the digital nomad lifestyle, living in and visiting different states/countries until she finds a permanent home again.

Website: www.jerralatrice.com
Instagram: @Childfree_Jerra
YouTube: @Childfree_Jerra
TikTok: @Childfree_Jerra

Notes from Cameron

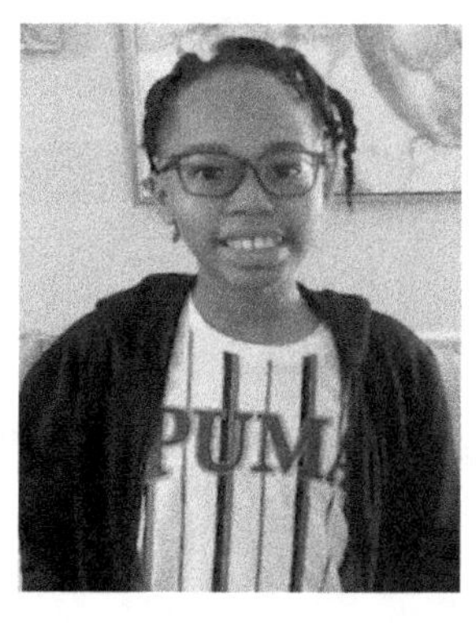

I am honored to have a chance to see this book early and proofread it. I liked how some parts were funny. I also like the confidence in this book, the opinions, and really everything about it.

To Arielle, I think you should really be a childfree activist. If you ever did a public speech about your life and choices, you would be the female Martin Luther King Jr. (but for childfree opinions, of course). I think you would kill it! Just, I didn't like it when you said how men reproduce. I really regretted looking up the meaning of that one word (orgasm).

Also, to my sweet and beautiful auntie, you're very creative with your book ideas. You're a really good author and should really get <u>MUCH</u> more recognition for your books, skills, passion, and creativity. To the readers reading this book and reached here, I appreciate you for getting this far, my auntie does too. Make sure you follow all the socials listed in this book too!

P.S. This is Jerra (again). I didn't know my nephew would add this, but I think it's cute..so I'm going to keep it.

Thanks for reading and be on the lookout for more books from me (possibly Cameron too)!